Positive

People

Positive People

Combating HIV and AIDS

Ian Mayo-Smith
Catherine Wyatt-Morley

Note for Librarians: A cataloguing record for this book is available from Library and Archives Canada at www.collectionscanada.ca/amicus/index-e.html
ISBN 1-4120-7662-5

TRAFFORD PUBLISHING™
Offices in Canada, USA, Ireland and UK

This book was published *on-demand* in cooperation with Trafford Publishing. On-demand publishing is a unique process and service of making a book available for retail sale to the public taking advantage of on-demand manufacturing and Internet marketing. On-demand publishing includes promotions, retail sales, manufacturing, order fulfilment, accounting and collecting royalties on behalf of the author.

Book sales for North America and international:
Trafford Publishing, 6E–2333 Government St.,
Victoria, BC V8T 4P4 CANADA
phone 250 383 6864 (toll-free 1 888 232 4444)
fax 250 383 6804; email to orders@trafford.com
Book sales in Europe:
Trafford Publishing (UK) Limited, 9 Park End Street, 2nd Floor
Oxford, UK OX1 1HH UNITED KINGDOM
phone 44 (0)1865 722 113 (local rate 0845 230 9601)
facsimile 44 (0)1865 722 868; info.uk@trafford.com
Order online at:
trafford.com/05-2557

10 9 8 7 6 5 4 3 2

Contents

Appendix

Acknowledgments

First we would both acknowledge George and Berni Lemon, who brought us together and who have been unfailing friends and supporters ever since. Then we cannot over-emphasize the part played in making this book possible by Ian's wife, Krishna Sondhi, publisher of Catherine's first book, "AIDS Memoir," and Catherine's three children all now grown and themselves parents. They have all been part of everything in this book.

All the clients of Women on Maintaining Education and Nutrition (W.O.M.E.N.) have made Catherine's life richer. Some of them have provided the basis for the stories in this book. Bishop George O. Adebanjo and his wife, Professor Adebanjo, have been a great source of support. We would also acknowledge our debt to all those who have at one time or another been members of the Executive Board of W.O.M.E.N.

Dr. Geeta Pfau at Eastern Connecticut State University, whose international work in combating HIV and AIDS on college campuses has earned her recognition, has been a valuable ally. In Thailand Dr. Somsak Chunharas opened many doors for us.

The developmental editorial skills of Ellis Whitman have been of great benefit to Catherine in the writing of the stories she tells in this book.

We thank you all for your invaluable help, but the remaining faults are all our own.

About the Authors
Brother and Sister

We are not really alike. One of us is male, the other female. One of us is black, the other white. One of us was born in the U.S., the other is a naturalized citizen. One of us is old enough to be the parent of the other. The are many other differences between us, but the one that matters for the purpose of this book is that one of us is HIV positive and the other is negative. (The one who is negative takes handfuls of pills every day for a heart condition. The one who is positive cannot take the pills she needs, because she has been deprived of her medical insurance.)

Yes, we both know how great a difference there is in our backgrounds and our present circumstances, and there's no biological connection between us, yet we know in our hearts that we are brother and sister. Neither of us thinks the other is perfect or anywhere near perfection, but our affection for each other is deep, long lasting and genuine.

How we came to get together has already been told by Catherine in her book *AIDS Memoir*. How all this has affected Ian is told below.

Inevitably some of our readers are going to ask "Are they romantically involved?" In this day and age such questions automatically pop into people's minds thanks to all the popular supermarket check out counter magazines and the TV programs that thrive on celebrity gossip. Well, we're sorry if it disappoints you, but we'd like to make it clear that though we love each other dearly we are not, have never been, and will never be romantically involved. One of us is happily married. The other currently single. But we are involved with each other in a thousand other ways, because we are brother and sister.

In many ways this is really Catherine's book. After the successful publication of *AIDS Memoir* Catherine continued writing and she had completed another large manuscript to be called "Time on the Path." She spent time on having it extensively edited. (Catherine is dyslectic and what she writes needs extra care in editing.) But she had not been able to find a publisher. Ian meanshile was continuing to write the socially aware poetry that he has published in his previous books of verses and essays and in the quarterly *The Lilypad* which he edited for six years. He suggested they do a book together. This is the result.

In this book all the stories except for "A Life Lived with a Mission," "Drinking, Drugs, HIV and My Life", and "Tommy Morris' were written by Catherine. Catherine also compiled the Appendix. "Drinking, Drugs, HIV and My Life" was written by Catherine's son, Aaron Welsh and has been previously published in *The Lilypad*. The rest, including all the poems, was written by Ian. A few of the poems have previously appeared in *The Lilypad*.

A Life Lived with a Mission

There it was, a large box about one foot high. It had come to me in my capacity as Vice Chairman of Kumarian Press. I opened it and found it full of papers, including an incredibly lengthy manuscript, a load of newspaper cuttings, and a videotape. Lets deal with the easiest thing first, I thought. I put the videotape into my video player and watched it. It was very moving. I phoned my wife, who is President and Publisher of Kumarian Press and told her, "You've got to see this." She too found it very moving. After that there was nothing to it but to start going through the rest of the mass of papers in the box. It took me about four days.

The box had come from Nashville from somebody I had never heard of. A covering letter from the sender told me how she had met a woman in the dentist's office. She got talking to this lady, a retired nurse, and told her that she had recently been in hospital for a hysterectomy and, while there, had been informed that she was infected with the HIV virus. She had been shocked as she was a married woman who had been faithful to her husband. He, alas, had been less than faithful and also had addictions to alcohol and other things, and he had infected her. She told the retired nurse that she had been writing a journal to leave behind for her children as she did not expect to live long. With the help of some other HIV positive people she had made a video. She asked if her new friend and her husband, a retired doctor, would care to see it.

So they came to a public showing of the video and were impressed by it. They also told her that they had friends in the publishing business (my wife and me) and they encouraged her to send us her manuscript. So that was how the box ended up on my desk.

The manuscript was an absolute mess and completely unpublishable as it was, but in it there were nuggets of pure gold. As you've no doubt guessed by now the manuscript had come from my co-author Catherine Wyatt-Morley. I talked to my wife, Krishna Sondhi, about it and we decided that, although it would involve a great deal of work, it could after extensive editing be turned into a really good book.

I went to Nashville, where my friends, Dr. George Lemon and his retired nurse wife, Bernice, lived and they kindly offered to put me up. I got to meet and talk with Catherine and her three children. I took some photos which ended up in the book. I was impressed with Catherine's amazing spirit. Eventually in 1997 Kumarian Press published Catherine's book *AIDS Memoir: Journal of an HIV Positive Mother.*

We stayed in regular touch by telephone and met whenever our paths crossed as they did in various parts of the U.S. I learned more about her.

I learnt that she had been a supervisor in the factory of a major industrial company - one of the largest in the U.S. if not the world. She and her husband had good incomes, a beautiful home, and a very comfortable lifestyle. I learnt how she had lost her job with the company as she became infected. I learnt how the company's medical office had broken all the rules of medical ethics by informing her workmates that she was infected. I learnt how she had lost her health insurance. I lerned how she was rejected and made unwelcome by her priest. But never, ever did I find that her spirit was broken. In fact sometimes I would phone her when I was feeling down and she would cheer me up. We spent a lot of time laughing together.

Since then I have vicariously lived through the difficulties she has had from time to time with her teenaged children. I have seen her build from scratch a community organization to support people, but particularly woman, who have been infected with or affected by the HIV virus and AIDS. I served as Vice Chair of the organization's board for several years. I have watched her as she coped with losses of funding for her organization. I have rejoiced with her as we attended her daughter's high school graduation. Although I was for years a professor at a state university, it is Catherine who has been my teacher regarding HIV and AIDS

I have a second home in Thailand and for seven years I taught project management to Thai officials, so I still have a number of contacts with senior Thai government people. I invited Catherine to come out to Thailand and stay at our home in Pattaya. She was there about a month. The first week she took a much needed rest, interspersed by intensive shopping forays. Thailand is a wonderful place to shop! But then we headed for Bangkok and I was able to introduce Catherine to senior officials in the Ministry of Public Health and the United Nations AIDS program. To say the least they were impressed with Catherine and all that she had to say. I had known already that she has the knack of gripping her audience's attention, whether that audience consists of one or two people or a crowd. She has since then been on trips to West Africa and to Switzerland, educating her listeners about HIV and AIDS and advocating the measures that need to be taken.

Catherine does not mince her words when she speaks. She really does tell it like it is. There are no taboo subjects when she comes to speak. At one time she came to a party at our house and I noticed that a number of the guests, particularly young women, seemed to have disappeared. So had Catherine. I found them in the kitchen where Catherine was holding forth to an apparently enthralled group of our guests on the subject of the dangers of becoming infected through oral sex.

Catherine continues to work with a vigor, a passion, and a faith, even though I have also seen the progress that the disease has made on her, with the steady falling of her T cell count, and her becoming prone to opportunistic infections. Just about everyone who featured in that original videotape that sparked my interest in Catherine and her work have died, but Catherine's determination and faith have kept her very much alive. Catherine, though a victim, resolutely refuses to act like one.

As I well know from my own and other people's experience, co-authoring a book can be a difficult business. It sometimes results in the breaking-up of a long-standing friendship. Egoes can get in the way.

Decisions like, whose name should come first on the front cover and title page can be fought over. But Catherine has been the best possible co-author. Whatever feelings of ego Catherine may have are totally subordinated to her determination to get the facts about HIV and AIDS as widely known as possible. Her dearest wish is to see this scourge brought under control and to end the terrible waste of human lives that is causing misery to millions around the world including so many children, who have been orphaned at an early age. So our names appear side by side on the front cover. Neither one is above the other.

I am proud to have such a wonderful sister to share life with. Catherine Wyatt-Morley embodies the concept of living positively.

Note. *Copies of "AIDS Memoir" are available from the publisher, Kumarian Press, Inc 1294 Blue Hill Avenue, Bloomfield, CT 06002 (toll free tel 800 289-2661) or from the organization that Catherine set up, W.O.M.E.N. (Women on Maintaining Education and Nutrition) 460 10th Circle North, Nashville TN 37203 (tel 615 256-3882.)*
Kumarian Press's website is ***www.kpbooks.com*** *and WOMEN's is* ***www.aidsnwomen.com.***

Unwelcome Revelation

I think my life is ended.
I just found out today
I'm broken, can't be mended.
That's all that I can say.

I wanted life insurance,
Had a physical exam.
It tested my endurance.
The doctor shut up like a clam.

We need, he said, to have a little chat.
I need to talk to you.
I wondered just what he was at.
I didn't have a clue.

He said, "Sit down, for what I say
May give you quite a scare."
So feeling this was not my day,
I sat down in a chair.

"We did some blood tests, as you know.
I just got the results today.
I'm afraid that this will be a blow.
You're blood is not OK.

"Tests showed a virus, HIV,
And as you know that's bad.
So now we must discuss with you
The treatments to be had."

I shook with shock, my head was reeling.
How could this thing be?
And then came this appalling feeling
My husband had infected me.

Don't be scared of me

I am not a leper.
You need not be scared of me.
You can come close to me
And you will not in any way be harmed.
In fact even though you don't know it,
You see me every day.
Every time you travel on the subway,
I am riding in the same car as you.
Every time you go to the supermarket
I will be shopping there.
When you go to church or temple
I am there in the congregation.
I am black and I am white.
I am Christian, Jewish, Muslim, Hindu and Buddhist.
I am a member of your extended family.
I am gay, straight, and bisexual.
I am a member of the armed forces and the police.
I am a teacher, a mechanic, an engineer,
A financial adviser, a bus driver.
I have served you meals in a restaurant
And I have cooked for you.

You are perfectly safe from me,
Unless, of course, you want to have sex with me.
But even that can be OK as long as you love me
And I am upfront with you about my condition.
But beware of me if I have sex with you
And do not tell you who I am,
For I am HIV infected
And I am everywhere.

Spirit of a Concubine

Elizabeth was a young blond with a slender build, she was a beautiful teenager filled with promise and passion. As a young child she daydreamed under the trees in the fields near her rural home about becoming an attorney and like most kids her age she hung out at the movie theater and the hamburger joint with her friends on weekends and during school breaks. She went to school dances and attended field trips with classmates. Her nightmare began at thirteen when her father, drunk as usual, sold her to a man whom she had never met. When the man came to the door to collect her, Elizabeth didn't understand what was happening, but her mother's tear-filled eyes told her she had to go with him.

Elizabeth was thrust into a world of beatings, verbal abuse, punishment, and unwanted sexual encounters with her keeper. The man, Aidis, was streetwise, twice her age, and a heavy drinker who used drugs. He supported them by gambling, and he was good at it. He gambled every night and his luck was admirable; he could outwit the most experienced gambler around and boasted about his skills to all. Aidis was small-time, though, a gambler who was too apprehensive to venture beyond the region - he never went for the big pay off. Elizabeth described him to me as being tall and slender, a blue-eyed, blond man with dark skin. She explained that the reason that Aidis gambled was to support his drug habit. He planned to strike it rich. To his buddies, he was arrogant and boastful, but at home his insecurity, and his heavy use of drugs, caused him to abuse Elizabeth mercilessly. Everything she did was wrong, yet when she begged him for her freedom, he told her that he never gave anything away.

As the abuse continued Elizabeth aged, her face was drawn and her flesh was bruised and battered. Now fifteen, she began shooting up heroin and became hooked. Now addicted, she shared dirty needles with Aidis and his gambling buddies. She also had sex with most of them, although she could seldom recall with whom. Elizabeth's world was out of control; the little girl with bright eyes had faded. During moments of sanity she would recall her dreams of assisting others as a lawyer. Visions danced through her mind - courtroom scenes where she saved the underdog while delivering justice, righting the wrongs of the justice system. Elizabeth's fantasies became more intense as she became more addicted to drugs and despair. Forced into prostitution to help pay for drugs and gambling debts, Elizabeth's nights were spent selling her body. After having sex with strangers for money, late at night, as she lay in her bed she dreamed of happier days. Anger would suddenly overwhelm her plummeting her backwards towards the stench of her reality, as feelings of abandonment and hatred toward the parents would seep through. Now, family was the needle and getting high was an elixir that allowed her to escape reality. She became increasingly dependent on Aidis, which only served to inflate his already enlarged ego. Now when he beat her and she didn't flinch, she felt useless and encapsulated, accepting any and all things he gave her. Like a wounded bird Elizabeth sold herself for her habit. A habit not chosen but based in her father's addiction to gambling and her mother's unwillingness to fight for her daughter.

With each morning her reality was washed in abandonment, abuse, drugs, the streets, men, and a haze filled head. Tormented she received the news of her mother's death from breast cancer in a letter from her father. Almost illiterate, she fought to read the words. Her father's letter was brief but she realized he had known where she was all those years and that if he knew where she was her mother knew where she was. The news of her mother's death last April brought so much pain that she couldn't cry. It was like the ice of her heart poured on the hot pavement of memories. She thought they didn't know she sold herself. Over time, Aidis told her the details of the deal with her father. No contract held her father to the deal and in drunken abusive rages he would say to her, "I bought you fair and square. Your family doesn't want you. If they did your Daddy wouldn't have gambled you away and your momma wouldn't have let you go. I'm a better man than your father. You're my slave, my concubine, my hoer, my bitch."

Everything Elizabeth experienced before her life changed seemed so far away. Between ages thirteen and sixteen, what was once a bright mined wishful thinking child, had grown to believe Aidis words.

Then Elizabeth remembered the lump under

her left arm. For months she had felt it but after learning of her mother's breast cancer she began to think of the lump. She had no insurance and never went to a doctor because Aidis didn't believe in them. If ever she was sick from a cold, or from a reaction to bad drugs, he would lock her in her room until she was well enough to do his bidding. One time she had had a bad reaction to some cocaine Aidis's buddy had gotten for her; to remedy this they made her drink a bottle of NyQuil. For days afterwards she lay in her own vomit, feces, and urine while Aidis yelled at her to clean herself up. Gathering strength she forced herself beyond human reasoning to eliminate all the drugs, legal and illegal, from her system.

One day when Aidis was away gambling she went to the free clinic and reported the lump under her left arm. She told the friendly nurse that her mother had died of breast cancer, and, as the words came out of Elizabeth's mouth, she realized it was the first time she had told anyone about her mother. She had not shared the letter or her father's news with Aidis. The nurse listened carefully, taking down each word and Elizabeth told her about her father's gambling her away, her drug use and prostitution, and the beatings from Aidis. She told her of how she had prayed for death to escape the torment. The weight of Elizabeth's words ripped at the nurse's heart. After fifteen minutes of talking the nurse suggested Elizabeth be seen by the clinic doctor. She assured her the doctor was nice and would help her. Reluctantly Elizabeth agreed after the nurse promised not to leave her. The doctor examined her finding old bruises, blood shot eyes, a vaginal infection, low blood pressure, a lump under her left arm. Needle tracks on her arms, between her toes and behind her knees stood out like solders ready for battle. He recommended having tests to determine what the lump was and suggested a blood test for levels of drugs in her system and an AIDS test, as well as a vaginal exam. He had given her cream to insert twice daily. Elizabeth was exhausted from the infection, emptied from using her body to support a habit she hated and drained from life.

Three weeks later she kept her scheduled appointment at the clinic. The nurse greeted her again and the two spent a few minutes talking. Elizabeth was comfortable with the nurse and felt that her secrets were safe with her. Things at home had gotten worse, Aidis had been having bad luck and money was tight. He was angry and had refused to give her money for food, so she was forced to sell herself since she had been to the clinic. The doctor had suggested she not have sexual contact in order to clear up the vaginal infection and alleviate some of the tearing he had found on her uterus and vaginal wall. With the return of her blood test Elizabeth was told she needed a biopsy and further testing to determine the extent of the lump. She was also told she had AIDS.

Elizabeth didn't know what to make of what the doctor said to her. She tried to clear her head but began to look to the nurse for help. The nurse held her hand with tears in her eyes and the room fell quiet. After a moment or two the doctor interrupted the silence by saying, "Elizabeth, we will do everything we can to help you, but you have to work with us. You need medical attention. I have a friend at the hospital downtown that is a cancer specialist. I'll give him a call today to see if he will work you in for free. I'll also recommend an infectious disease specialist friend who will help you cope with AIDS. Do you know what AIDS is Elizabeth?"

"No, not really. I have heard of it," she replied.

Elizabeth didn't move for a long moment, then the nurse told her that she would help her get dressed as well as help her get to the appointments.

"Just let us help. I care," the nurse said.

Elizabeth was silent but her mind focused on Aidis. What would he say if she told him? Should she tell him? Would he let her get medical attention? Would he beat her if she told him? Did Aidis give her AIDS? The doctor stepped out of the room to arrange the appointments. Elizabeth and the nurse were alone in the room. It was as if the nurse could read her mind.

"When will Aidis be home?" the nurse asked.

"Tomorrow night."

"OK that gives you until then to get your things."

"What do you mean, get my things?"

"You are coming to live with me," said the nurse.

Elizabeth nodded in relief and agreement.

One morning my telephone rang. It was Elizabeth.

"Hello Catherine, my name is Elizabeth. My

doctor gave me your telephone number and suggested I call. I hope you don't mind."

"No Elizabeth, I don't mind at all," I said.

After a long moment she said, "My doctor told me about you. He said you help girls with AIDS."

We talked for a long time. I understood her confusion. On the telephone, Elizabeth sounded so young, and, as we spoke, I thought of my own daughter. Elizabeth had been through so much suffering. I was glad to hear that she had a supportive medical team who had helped her get through a diagnosis of AIDS. The lump under Elizabeth's left arm had been diagnosed and she was now in chemotherapy and had already undergone surgery to remove the lump.

We arranged a meeting place, and from that point on Elizabeth and I grew to become women with a common goal. She told me all about her life and how she had been dealing with AIDS, cancer, and chemotherapy. She had moved from the rural town where she had lived. Elizabeth had left Aidis and had not looked back. The concubine was finally free and had moved in with the nurse for a while but eventually, after making friends, had found an apartment with a roommate. Elizabeth had begun putting her life in order and took on a fresh perspective. I counseled her regularly and became her friend and mentor. I shared my own story with her and told her about my children and my family. Elizabeth, now an empowered young woman, had beaten the odds. She gambled and found people do care.

With the help she received Elizabeth succeeded in beating the odds and found a life. The daughter of my next door neighbor in Thailand was les fortunate.

Death of a Peasant Girl in Thailand

There were no flowers,
Not even chairs for the mourners to sit on.
She came from a poor family.
There was no money for likay performances
And she could only be laid for two days
In the funeral hall
Before the cremation,
So this was a cut price funeral,
The best her family could do.
But she is missed.
There is much sadness.
She was only twenty seven, I am told,
And left behind a little girl of ten.
It was her husband who infected her.
He's still alive, though she has died.
Death from AIDS
Can be very ugly as well as painful
In body and in mind.
She had been a pretty girl.
She laughed and smiled a lot,
Though she never had much
Except her little girl.
May her rest free her from pain.
And may her daughter find comfort,
Though I know not whence it can come.
Some pains like HIV are incurable.

James - Broken Hearted

On Tuesday a man named James, a single parent to a teenage daughter, came to see me. His wife, a nurse, had died of AIDS three years prior. James, a middle-aged man with a great sense of humor, a strong personality and a great love for his daughter had a style of his own. His concern for his daughter, as the single parent of a teenage girl whose mother had passed away, was tangible. His wife had been ill for a long time and her illness took its toll on James and their daughter. Taking care of his ailing wife meant working full time, cooking the meals that no one seemed to eat, cleaning a house that was never clean, picking up their daughter from school, teachers' conferences, hospital stays, and administering medications.

Although James and his daughter are both HIV negative, he is concerned about his daughter having unprotected sex.

He said, "I know what I was doing, or trying to do, at her age. Now kids can get more than pregnant."

I told James, "I think our society has lost many of its morals, finding self-gratification more important than anything else does."

He agreed and explained that his daughter had retreated after her mother's death. Bitterness, anger, and rejection are her moods most often, he confesses.

He confided, "I just want to shake her sometimes. Her mouth at times is more than I can handle."

"Yes, James I have one of those myself," I comforted him.

James's wife had contracted the virus from a patient. All precautions had been in place and she prided herself on using them. After she had suffered a puncture wound from an unsterilized needle, the staff went into overdrive, rinsing soaping, and desperately scrubbing the affected area. These precautions did not prevent her from becoming HIV positive. The time before she received the news was excruciating. Wondering if she would test positive, praying she would test negative. Time passed, and as the disease gripped she lapsed into AIDS all too soon. During those months James his wife and their daughter fought for her survival, but to no avail. They grew closer as a family, spending time loving one another's company. Those moments are captured in his heart and I could see a light behind his eyes as he spoke fondly of that special time. His wife died of an AIDS-related opportunistic infection.

Since then James has become a full-time single parent. He had to deal with his wife's death and the many issues that it has left their daughter with.

"My daughter's faith in God was replaced by anger," he said. "She has become rude, untrusting, all the while blaming everyone else for the pain she felt. Before, during, and after the funeral she shut down and was angry with a dead person, her own mother, for leaving her. How could she understand?"

In the time between events that led to the death of his wife, James had to figure out how to love his daughter, yet not allow her to be destroyed by her pain. I think he's still trying to figure that one out.

Understanding James, I could only tell him of my own experience with my two boys and my daughter.

"Living with an HIV positive activist mother does not mean my children always make the right decisions. After all they are teenagers, too. I am certainly a proactive mother speaking to them about any and all things. As parents it is important to give your children all the tools necessary to make an informed decision," I said. "After that parents have prayer. It is their responsibility to use those tools. A wounded child lashes out at authority."

James nodded his head in agreement.

With discussion, spirituality, parental guidance, and love children will begin to recognize that the injustice of a parent's illness or death is not that, or the other parent's, fault. A single parent can become the only stable person left to be angry at. The problem is dealing with those teenage years. It is tragic to witness the pain of children and be unable to do anything except comfort them through it. With my own teens I have found it important to give them love above all, as much stability as possible, a sense of always being there for them, and a spiritual base.

AIDS often leaves a child, like James's daughter, missing one or both parents. If the child is lucky he or she may have grandparents to take over the parental role. But this is not easy on either the child or the grandparents

Grandparent

When I reached the age of sixty-five
I quit my job, retired and thought
I'm glad to be alive
And so I bought
A little place where Anne and I
Could just relax and watch the world go by,
But little did I know
How short a time would go
Before our lives would change
And we would have to completely rearrange
The comfortable retirement we had planned,
For our world got completely out of hand
When AIDS took our daughter Kate away.
Her husband died some months earlier, by the way.
Kate's death was tragedy enough, as you'll agree
But now we've her teenage children, not one, but three,
Who we have to bring up and educate.
We never could have foreseen that this would be our fate.
We love our grandkids dearly,
But they are very clearly
At a very problematic stage of life,
And even simple discipline can lead to strife.

We want them to grow up healthy and strong
With a clear knowledge of right and wrong.
Able to make right choices,
But sometimes we hear their voices
Whining, complaining, full of rebellion.
Our patience is sorely tried by the little hellion.
We know they're all good kids at heart,
But it can be awfully difficult for us to play our part.

Despite all the information that is now available about HIV and AIDS, many people all over the world continue to play Russian roulette with their sex lives.

Russian Roulette

This girl who lies beside me in my bed
Is holding a gun to my head.
We are playing Russian roulette.
I know I am not infected
At least no virus was detected
Last time I went for a test,
So I hope all's for the best,
But in fact the sexual history
Of the girl I'm with is a mystery
And we're both playing Russian roulette.
But the trigger, we're going to pull it
And we pray in the chamber's no bullet.

Cheryl - Reasons To Live

When Cheryl came by the office one afternoon I found her to be a fragile woman searching for reasons to live. She had been in therapy for two and a half years but had not progressed and her psychologist had run out of insurable sessions. Her therapist made suggestions and had even gone so far as to administer rapid eye movement therapy, but Cheryl felt she had come to a crossroads. Her therapy, was in her own word, "useless." She sought to find the turning point that would free her to heal.

Cheryl couldn't move forward and leave behind her feelings of low self-esteem and hollowness about her diagnosis. Cheryl had been diagnosed HIV positive shortly before her husband committed suicide. He deliberately ran off the road and killed himself very soon after their diagnoses. He couldn't handle the news of being infected and having infected the woman he loved so much. Cheryl and her husband had been deeply demoralized and downhearted, they spoke only of the many negative aspects of HIV/AIDS. There was hopelessness on the road ahead of them, and he begged her for forgiveness, not listening to her forgiving words.

They discovered that he was infected when they received a phone call from a Red Cross representative who notified them that he needed to come in to discuss a discrepancy found in his blood. Cheryl had taken the phone demanding reasons for her husband's appearance at the Red Cross. The spokesperson gave her little information but eventually suggested they both see their family doctor. "Results can be sent to your doctor," said the voice on the other end of the telephone.

By the time they arrived at their doctor's office the Red Cross had faxed the report. Their doctor suggested they take an HIV test. They agreed reluctantly. Ten days later the results were positive for them both. Immediately Cheryl's husband plunged into a deep depression, and, with no one to talk to, Cheryl followed suit. In no way were they prepared to attend support groups, tell friends, family, or coworkers. The pain became greater as time elapsed, and yet they suffered in silence. Cheryl knew she needed psychological help. She suggested they go together, but he refused. Cheryl phoned their doctor to get the name of a psychologist in the area. She made an appointment for the next day. As Cheryl sought therapy for her sanity, her husband froze. Paralyzed, his doors to sanity closed. He had gone underground abandoning their love in attempts to escape HIV/AIDS. What was once a loving, trusting relationship became cold and lonely for them both. They were living in the same house, but the division between them, was in Cheryl's words, "wider than the Grand Canyon." Cheryl's sessions with the psychologist had given her a place to go twice a week but little else. She knew she needed something more.

She stopped by to see me because a friend had attended one of my lectures. They had met in front of Cheryl's psychologist's office one evening as the friend was on her way to hear me speak. Having read my book, Cheryl's friend handed it to her saying, "Read this. She's been through hell and now I am going to hear about how she came back and what motivates her to go on." Cheryl's friend was unaware of her HIV status. She called her friend the next day and asked how the meeting went. Her friend told her how frank I had been, speaking freely about real issues.

Cheryl told me she took the book home and didn't put it down until she was done reading it. Crying, laughing, agreeing, and getting mad, Cheryl read and filled her spirit. She told me that after she finished reading it she had decided that she had to meet me.

My conversations with Cheryl were profound. She had many questions about personal things not printed in the book. It was during these conversations, over time, that I began to see empowerment sprout in her. She told me she hadn't felt that much relief since before being diagnosed. Over a cup of tea a few weeks after our first meeting with tears and sobs Cheryl recalled the tragic death of her husband. She detailed their relationship and the emptiness he had left. He had left her leaving her to grieve his death in anguish. Cheryl mourned her husband. Understanding her feelings, I shared my aloneness with her. We comforted each other, and the moment hung in the air like music. We shared the bridge to hope and the pain of diagnosis, as well the fear of death and dying, and the reality of loss.

At Cheryl's request I shared events of my four

years working and growing within the ACTG/CCG, (AIDS Clinical Trails Group/Community Constituency Group),the Patient Care Committee, and the Women's Committee and the Adult Executive Community. She was interested to know what goes on within government bodies allocating funds for research. She wanted to know where research is heading and where exactly the cure is: "Is there a cure? What happens at these meetings? Tell me about it."

Refilling my cup of tea and turning to Cheryl, I recalled my first much anticipated executive community meeting. I had finally made it to the top and had an arena to push women's health issues, or so I thought. The first meeting I attended with the ACTG Adult Executive Community was awfully disappointing, I told her. The only woman of color, and the new kid on the block, I sat in a corner listening to the debates of leading researchers and doctors argue for over an half an hour about whose name would be placed first on a position paper or some such document. I sat there looking at my watch, horrified to witness their priorities. Each researcher (principle investigator) gave his opinion on why their name should appear first citing all their hard work and that of his staff. After arguments were heard there was a vote. One became disgruntled and left the meeting in a huff after his opponent won the vote. Discussion about the issues that brought us there was limited due to time. In some of those discussions there was talk of de-funding ACTG sites for not reaching set goals and for other reasons that were unclear to me. In disbelief I walked out of my first meeting wondering, was this all? Surely somebody was doing something. It was the beginning of bureaucracy on a different level.

On Cheryl's next visit with me she asked me to pick up the conversation with my experience with the CCG. I glanced toward the ceiling, recalling to Cheryl the years of struggle to get a sound women's agenda included in clinical trials past the CCG. At the time few trials were conducted for women and the research was dramatically behind. The only three women of color, myself included, relentlessly fought for women's rights. Sadly some CCG representatives continue to harbor rifts between a "gay white male agenda" and a "women's health agenda." This fragmentation fractures the mission and purpose of the CCG, splitting the result. Important agenda ideals have been surprisingly crushed, tabled, or held up, and equal access to technology has not consistently been in place.

Since the gay community was ravished by HIV/AIDS in the beginning of the epidemic their community has suffered extensively. The gay community faced tremendous loss and fought with government leadership, including President Ronald Reagan, and a scientific community not knowing how to deal with the "gay plague." Progression of AIDS over the first decade in the gay community has brought experience, mobilization, awareness, a demand for addressing treatment, drugs, care and a network. These skills are to be recognized and commended. However the face of AIDS has changed and the need for equal representation is apparent. The "in-fighting" within the Community

Constituency Group (CCG) at times was overwhelming. Cheryl sat in amazement, forgetting her worries as I shared the need for pushing a strong women's agenda within the CCG/ACTG.

In memory I took Cheryl back to the meeting in which Community Advisory Board (CAB) members and Act Up supporters stormed a CCG meeting demanding equal community representation sighting failure after failure within the ACTG/CCG. In addition to this they were angry that principle investigators showed a lack of support in the community's concerns within the clinical setting and the fact that ACTG sites did not provide consistent treatment, thus resulting in inequality of service.

During another encounter Cheryl and I turned our attention to the more personal aspects of an HIV positive woman. Though not considering getting into any relationship Cheryl asked how infected women are coping with HIV/AIDS and how they find it within themselves to have relationships after diagnosis. She said, "I feel like damaged goods." She couldn't conceive being in a relationship since it was a man who brought her to this point. I decided to share the experience of a friend living in Los Angeles. Tamara and her significant other had found love and trust, they share a warm and sexual relationship. They practice safe sex and enjoy each other. For them it's more about being together and sharing love on a deeper level than that sex offers. It is one that Tamara never expected but one she is grateful for. She says "Hell, I am more honest because what do I have to lose?" Tamara was forced into prostitution after running away from home. Hindsight had shown her that her home wasn't so bad, but prostitution had damaged her soul, and Tamara's self-esteem was low when she was admitted into a halfway house. It was during that time she found a man who showed continuing support, concern, then love. They've been together ever since and both are better people for having the other in their life.

Looking forward, Cheryl's shoulders began to straighten as I told her that women with HIV are having relationships, getting married, and finding love. I reminded her of the importance of honesty and disclosing to potential partners. It can be a gamble, but not disclosing is criminal, not to mention immoral. Cheryl felt better after our conversations, but I knew it was only a distraction from her reality. She admitted to needing more conversations with her psychologist as well. Each week Cheryl came to talk to me she became taken-up in possibilities. She began to seek me as a guide to crossing over into reasons to live, someone to heal the emotional and physical wounds her husband had created both in life and in death.

Cheryl poured out her violation, betrayal, and humiliation in a shower of pain. She brought to our conversations emotional baggage too heavy to carry alone. She occupied my mind with her anger. Cheryl said, "Did you know people are now infecting one another intentionally, using AIDS as a weapon of warfare?" Over time Cheryl began to recognize that she could only change herself and had no control over people or her past. She needed to come to terms with her emotions before she could come to terms with HIV/AIDS. She doesn't believe her husband infected her intentionally, but her husband is not around to answer those questions.

No one should ever condemn prostitutes or (to use the euphemism) sex workers out of hand, unless they know the whole story of how they come to be living as they do. Many young women in Thailand and other poorer countries are driven into this trade. Their chances of being infected are very high, like the girl Lek whose story is below.

Lek

Her age was nineteen and her name was Lek.
She had little education but what the heck!
She had learned to listen or pretend she did
But what her feelings were she hid.
She worked at the bar called The Lucky Monkey
Where the music they played was loud and funky.
The farangs* came there with their thirst and their lust
And she went with them as she knew she must.

He came into the bar at nine,
Looked around, saw her, paid her bar fine,
So that he could take her out.
He was European, bald and stout.
He was about three times her age
And she was just another page
In the mental diary that he kept.
Jesus wept.

At least he saw that she was fed
Before he took her to his hotel bed,
But it did not make her feel very good
When he said she could only have Thai food,

For farang food cost too much money
To spend on his temporary honey.
He led her holding her arm tight
As if afraid she might get out of sight
And run away.
Oh, Lord we pray.

Does she really believe it is her karma
To play a pathetic role in this earthly drama,
Men versus women, rich versus poor
In an unending, unstoppable war?
But no, she still has hope
Someone will rescue her from the slippery slope
On which she's sliding down.
He'll be a farang who will smile, not frown,
And he will love her, want her for his wife
And take her far away from this her present life.

But it is clear he has not come tonight
So she must put on a face that's bright,
Pretending everything's all right
Till he has satisfied his appetite
And lets her go. Tomorrow is another day
Perhaps the pain and shame will go away.
And so she pays her sad life's tolls.
Oh, Lord have mercy on our souls.

* *A farang is a Western foreigner in Thailand*

Charlie - Talk with the Junk Yard Dog

Charlie called me one night when he found my card at a local truck stop.

"Hey, I hear you talk to people who have this AIDS thing," he shouted into the phone.

"Yes I do," I said.

"Well, let me tell you, lady, there are lots of us out here with nowhere to go, no food, and no place to sleep. This AIDS thing means nothing when you're trying to eat. I ride my bike all over the country and run across teenagers living in abandoned train cars that haven't seen home in years. They're all ages and come in all colors. You know what I mean?"

"Yes, I do," I said.

"These kids are running from jail, they're running from mommies and daddies who beat 'em, and they have more drugs than even I can do," he shouted.

Charlie went on to say, "But most of them are good kids. They're out here not 'cause they want to be but 'cause they have nothing to go back to. You hear me?"

"Yes, I'm listening, Charlie," I said.

I could tell Charlie needed to share his experience with me. He was not calling to get advice nor was he seeking information about HIV/AIDS; he was calling to give me advice. Charlie's advice was coming at a time shortly after a teenager I was very fond of had recently died of a drug-related overdose. I found what he said very interesting, hence I listened very intently, but unfortunately his words were all too familiar.

"Me, I can take care of myself, but you'd better do something about those kids out here. What do you suggest I do?"

"How can I help?" I asked him

"Get 'em some help find 'em a place to sleep. They don't care about having AIDS they just want a warm place. You can't get through to 'em about AIDS when they haven't got nothing to eat or a place to sleep."

"I know, Charlie. I'm a mother, and I thank God every day my kids are home and safe."

"Listen, lady, I don't have long. I have got to get going but I thought you should know."

"Know what, Charlie?" I queried.

"Listen, I fought for this country and it rips my heart out to see these young kids out here with nothing. Tell them administrator people we can't afford them pills they want us to take. Can you afford 'em?"

"No Charlie I can't afford them either." I went on to say, "Right now I'm not taking the medications, but soon I'll have no choice."

Worried about him, I asked, "Charlie, how are you? How are you surviving with AIDS and no medicine?"

"The same way you are, lady. One day at a time!"

On Charlie's end of the phone I could hear loud noises and dishes clanking. People were talking and I heard country music blaring, among many other sounds.

Charlie said, "Just a minute."

When he came back to the phone he said, "Well, the kids on the streets can't afford 'em, none of us can. Like I said, we have other stuff to deal with, but you can do something, lady. Them kids remind me of myself. They're young and could be somebody."

He went on to say, "I hear you got connections, so I'm tellin' you, do something."

"Charlie, I promise you I'm trying."

"OK, OK, lady, I didn't mean to get on you. I'm sure you're doin' your best."

"Oh, Charlie, I care deeply for those kids. I know what it's like to have this disease and have no one to talk to. My heart aches for the kids."

Charlie said, "Well, keep doin' whatever you're doin'."

He ended our conversation with, "I have got to go they're putting the trash out and that's my dinner. You'd be surprised what people throw away. Thanks for talkin', lady. I'll call you if I'm back this way again."

"Keep my card, Charlie, and let me know how you're doing. Take care, and thanks for calling."

The phone line went dead. My conversation with him stayed with me. I dreamed about him and those kids.

Charles Cannon, now known as "Charlie, the bicycle bum," carries everything he owns in saddlebags, which hang on either side of his bike, the rest of his worldly belongings wrapped in garbage bags stuffed in a basket draped on the handlebars. Charlie has AIDS. He is considered human garbage, a transient viewed as a lowlife and the scum of the earth. Charlie is a

Vietnam veteran with no place to call home. These days we step over or look at the Charlies of this world with distrust and downcast eyes, if we notice them at all. He travels the country trying to find something, unsure of what that something is.

If a lowlife bum like Charlie, a Vietnam veteran, has heart enough to show concern for the kids he sees on the streets each day, who are we to ignore the children? The fight for America's children is indeed enormous. The rates of infection among our youth are outrageous, but we can't give up. We could pin the blame on media, on music, or on parents, but that doesn't change the facts. Blame is useless in light of rates of continued infections. Who's talking to the children? How can we save the children? We have to get to each one. In the words of a dear friend who died of AIDS, "Reach one, teach one. They hear what you say, and they hear what you don't say."

Many of the women working in the sex trade would stand a much better chance of avoiding being infected if their customers would all wear condoms, but sometimes their customers lack both compassion and commonsense, like the one in the poem below,

Condom

She wants me to wear a condom?
Do I wear gloves when I wash my hands?
What nonsense is this?
Why should I wear a condom?
I'm paying her well
And I expect her to do as I wish.
If she wants me to wear a condom
Because she's infected,
Then forget the whole thing.
I'll find another girl who's clean.
I tell you I'm clean
And I've never worn a condom yet
And I don't intend to.
Is she afraid of getting pregnant?
Surely she's on the pill, isn't she?

Make up your mind, girl,
Do we go ahead or not?
I can't stand around all day
Or the effects of the Viagra may wear off.

In this country and many others the top sports stars are seen as role models by millions of young people. That's fine so long as they live accordingly, but unfortunately some of them prefer to take advantage of their fame and fortune in the worst way and are anything but good role models for young men and women. The very wealthy sports stars, if they do become infected are probably able to pay for the most expensive medical care, but the people they may infect are not likely to be wealthy and may totally lack health insurance.

The Magic Circle

Magic Johnson, I hear, says he's had a hundred women.
The art of seduction he's certainly perfected.
One of them must have infected him.
I wonder how many he's infected.

Ayina - African Sister

An African woman unique in her right. Ayina remained true to the heritage of her foremothers. She is yellow-skinned, and has coarse black hair and wide hips. This woman has known discrimination and suffered its effects. Her roots are blackened with the rightness of whiteness. The plague of institutionalized racism haunts every native African. To better herself she sacrificed much, traveling miles and living with strangers to finish school. Once high school was completed Ayina left her village; it was time for educating herself. University life was rich with knowledge, but graduation came too quickly. Settling into her medical duties brought much pain with the knowledge that she gained. She discovered her countryman filled the beds with disease. She knew that tuberculosis, herpes, and untreated sexually transmitted disease increased the risk of HIV. Her reality was that the life expectancy for her fellow Africans has decreased by five years, and one hundred percent of blood supplies are still not checked. Fifty percent of the hospitalized populations living in Africa suffer from illness associated with AIDS, and 1996 brought her African nation to realize 500,000 of her countrymen are now infected. The epidemic spread faster in this timeframe resulting in over 1.5 million people dead of AIDS. More than 8,500 new infections occurred daily and one thousand children under the age of fifteen became infected every day, most transmitted from mother to child. Of the remaining 7,500 new cases reported 40 percent are women.

Fifteen percent of these infections are occurring in young adults between the ages of fifteen and twenty-five. Ninety percent of new infections occur in developing countries worldwide. Modern medicines available in the west at a price unreachable by many westerners are not available for her population. Africa is a continent with a variety of cultures and traditions; what all African nations share is the AIDS crisis, which has impacted the health and economy of the continent. Regions south of the Sahara are densely populated with people who have AIDS, and today traffic accidents and cancer are now second and third to the losses of AIDS.

In Africa over 1,000,000 children are left orphaned by AIDS, and these motherless children huddle in hospital corridors waiting. Ayina saw first hand the powerlessness as the family and friends of deceased patients cried for their losses. Ayina knows that the AIDS children of this plateau must be cared for with more that mere aspirin. However, wiping tears is not her approach; rather Ayina remains steadfast and demanding. Writing letters, following protocols, e-mailing contacts in the west, and developing public services has gotten little result. When I met with her she slammed her fist on the desk in her closet sized office and exploded. "My people are becoming the disposable population. We are truly in this for the long haul, not an outbreak." Torn apart with rage, her blood boils rapidly as she recognizes the decimation of her people from the AIDS epidemic.

At night she has nightmares and by day she

treats babies, mothers, and her countrymen with little more than aspirin and antibiotics. Praying for technology, for the proper tools to fight the disease, Ayina knows that this won't solve all the problems. Getting proper health care to her area and other developing countries remains an uphill struggle. It's not enough to have the drugs, it's not enough to have the tests. Despite research and good intentions the epidemic accelerates. Money, training, new clinics, overcoming cultural stigmas, and reversing family thinking are just a few of the other issues haunting her thoughts. Ayina began creating a refuge for her countrymen with AIDS. Tirelessly she fights to make medications available. Together she and her mate disseminate prevention methods. Effective condom distribution and formulating education that is community based and interesting to the younger, more susceptible members of society is part of her fight. Collaboration with fellow doctors has enhanced her ability to treat her countrymen with more Western approaches while continuing with her cultural traditions and alternative heritage.

Ayina has a sister living in the Untied States. I met Obia at a dinner honoring HIV/AIDS volunteers. She was a very talkative lady. Seated at a front table, I asked about her accent and she told of moving to the United States with her husband. Her husband a doctor came to Tennessee to teach classes at Meharry Medical College. He was the host of the event and her reason for being there. They live in a remote area outside Nashville. She complained of feeling isolated and out of place. At the time of our meeting, Obia had not shared the news of her HIV infection with Ayina or any of her African family. Even though she lives in America now, Obia is unable to speak the words for fear of bringing family disgrace. In a deep African accent she spoke about life in Africa and her place in her family. Being the older daughter, she had not been able to attend school, but instead she worked as a maid to support her siblings. She spoke proudly of her sister Ayina.

Obia lost a child to AIDS since living in America, but AIDS was not discussed at the child's burial ceremony, which took place in their homeland. Another child was stillborn. The two sisters sat silent as their future generation was buried. Lives intertwined but truths were unshared. As she shared this intimate detail of her life with me I thought, shivers run through hearts that are burdened with more than death. Shame closes doors of family discussion and support.

Obia made sure I had got Ayina's e-mail address, and she and I have gotten to know one another through e-mails. Ayina was overjoyed to share with me the news of her pregnancy, but at the same time she felt a sense of foreboding with the idea of raising a child in a disease infected society. In America her sister, Obia, keeps silent. I visit her at home and discuss treatment and her reactions to the latest drug regiment, but she will not participate in women's groups or anything totally related to HIV/AIDS. Obia uses a P.O. box to receive any information about HIV/AIDS. She doubles, and even triple, bags her garbage in attempts to protect their privacy. Medical records and anything relating to her care have a PO box number. It is important to her that no one finds out. I respect her wishes and in doing so I see to it that her P.O. box is always used.

Obia knew I was writing a second book and told me how much she enjoyed the first one. *AIDS Memoir: Journal of an HIV Positive Mother* gave her comfort in part because she could read about women with HIV in the privacy of her own home and not feel uneasiness. I had given her a copy of the video "Reasons To Live: Women, Their Families, and HIV" as well. She shared the video with her husband who in turn took it to Meharry to share with his students. I had found getting to know Ayina through e-mail and Obia through ongoing visits to her home very enlightening. I wanted to write about her very much. When I asked Obia if I could write about her I was only allowed the privilege to share this small part of her life. I had to agree to change her name. Her story is important because it draws a clear portrait of the measures some woman must go through to keep quiet about HIV. There is more to Obia's story, but this small picture sheds lights on women of color, culture, pride, Africa, America, HIV positive children, isolation and so much more.

Ayina needs medicines to do her work effectiely, but she can't get them. Obia needs them for her own treatment. Why is it that only the lucky ones, who are either very well insured or wealthy can get the drugs they need, if they become infected?

Pharmaceuticals

Can someone tell me why
Drug prices are so high?
It's really past endurance
For I lost my insurance
Because I was infected
By a man whom I had respected.
You see I was his wife,
Yet he destroyed my life.

I need to have those pills
To counteract the ills
This dread disease has brought.
I never would have thought
An affluent woman that I was
Should suffer so much, just because
Of corporate greed
That does not care for need,
But rather would define
Their humanitarian mission by their bottom line.

If I had money and could go
To many other countries, there I know

I could buy these drugs at much less cost.
But I don't have that money, so I'm lost.
But could someone tell me, please,
Why they have to squeeze
People like me and don't let me buy
Those medicines at a price that I
Could just afford? I just abhor
To see their profits soar
While they leave me in despair.
Why don't they care?
Can it really be their only need
Is to satisfy their investors' greed?

Tina - What's love got to do with it?

A lady I will call Tina had been volunteering for a while. She and her husband led very interesting high-profile lives. Perry was an executive in charge of marketing at a fast-paced computer company, and Tina was a well-respected television anchor. They had no children by choice, and their home was filled with fifteen years of marital memories - sculptures, plants, and antiques were found throughout their million-dollar spread. At the time Tina was thirty-seven and Perry was thirty-nine, and they had captured the American dream. Business leaders came to unwind, relax, and party in their beautiful home. They smiled in public but behind closed doors they smoked crack cocaine and shared the sexual favors of strangers lapping up the pleasure of secrecy. Few knew that behind close doors Perry beat Tina once or twice a week, depending on how his week was going and the pressure he was under. Tina described his job as highly stressful, and very demanding, and his having to produce numbers by any means necessary.

Tina told me she loved her work, "It was the one thing that gave my life purpose. All the material things we had meant little to me, but my job kept me focused and gave me the determination to succeed." Late one warm summer evening Tina and Perry were hosting a party to celebrate a promotion and raise she had received at her job. Champagne filled the partygoers' glasses, the lavish spreads of food were by the finest catering service money could buy. That evening in

August while in the middle of the festivity, partygoers were startled by Perry's behavior. Perry had become agitated after smoking several pipes of crack in the downstairs bathroom during the evening. Storming through their assembled friends, Perry shouted obscenities over the music at Tina from across the room. He threw his scotch glass at her, demanding her attention to see the spider crawling up the wall. When she told him there was no spider on the wall, it further infuriated him. By then the last of their guests had left and suddenly the house was big and empty. Tina had not anticipated the rest of the night would change her life forever.

After dismissing the catering service staff, Tina went into the kitchen and began to clean nervously. Perry came into the kitchen and stood in the doorway starring at the walls, making comments about the bugs crawling on them. Tina said nothing, bypassing him and heading upstairs to their bedroom. Hallucinating about bugs, angry with her for embarrassing him in front of their friends, and mad that the bugs were now crawling on him, Perry followed her into the bedroom.

In the past Perry would remain in turmoil after beating Tina. But his promises to never hit her again faded as she pointed the 38 revolver at his chest on that night. It was a calm August summer evening and Tina had had enough. She pleaded with Perry as he tossed her about their bedroom like a rag doll. In the bedroom Tina's head landed near the nightstand where the gun was kept. Her life changed in that instant. Tina killed her husband. As she recalled it, “It's still a blur.”

Tina spent the next few years between jail and court and doing time for taking a life had taken its toll on her, Tina said. Much time behind bars passed slowly. Tina was sent to a halfway program for abused and battered woman. While there she befriended a woman named Alice who was dying of AIDS. Alice had suffered abuse from her live-in boyfriend, the father of her five children. He had also infected her. Alice found she was infected during the stillborn delivery of their sixth child. Tina and Alice were very different coming from different backgrounds, but the similarities were astonishing. At the halfway center, Tina spent time caring for HIV/AIDS patients like her friend Alice.

Eight years later Tina had become an important part of the center. Alice had died two years earlier of cervical cancer and Tina had taken her friend's death hard. Vowing to continue Tina grew as a person because the shallowness of her former existence had not allowed her to see how others lived. Alice had made a tremendous impact on Tina's life. But through the taking of her husband's life, even though it had been in self-defense, she had changed. Her time behind bars, together with volunteering in a setting where people depended on her, meant more than she knew.

By the time Tina came into my life her heart was softened, and volunteering for causes she believed in had indeed become her calling. Left well off without financial worry, Tina comes in as often as she can to file, do advocate work for abused and battered women, make follow-up telephone calls, and make sure my calendar is followed to the letter. Her work with Women On Maintaining Education and Nutrition is a gift.

In these days age is no longer a bar to sexual acticity, but we never hear much about HIV and AIDS among the elderly. All the same the infection is spreading amongst the elderly at an alarming rate.

AIDS and the elderly

No one likes to admit they're past it.
Sex is part of being alive.
Don't think you ever will outlast it.
That longing for intimacy will always thrive.

For male dysfunction there are all these drugs.
They'll soon have some for women too.
We'll not be contented just with hugs.
I want the full monty. Say, don't you?

Young folk don't seem to realize
That seniors are sexual people still.
It's not enough to idealize
Love. We want to experience the sensual thrill

We're not always as careful as we should be.
How could this granny be infected?
But AIDS spreads through the retirement community
In ways few people have suspected.

This infection does not discriminate
Against the elderly of any race.
It offers a horrendous end, so hesitate,
Take care and live your life with grace.

Heroin Addict

My arm is scarred with puncture marks.
I dread the questions of some narcs
About the source of my supply.
This shit's not working like it did before
But every day I need it more and more.
If I don't get some I will die.

I know about infected needles anyhow,
But I have to to have this shot right now.
Hey, lend me that! I need to shoot up too.
Don't warn me of the danger. I don't care.
I need it here and how, not then and there.
I'll do what this compulsion makes me do.

So what if I get infected, what the hell!
My life is hell already, can't you tell.
This smack is what makes it bearable at all.
Nothing could be worse than going without
This shit I put into my veins, no doubt,
And if I fall for HIV, well then I fall.

Jerry - Addiction conquered

The automotive industry has had an economic stronghold in Michigan for years. Building an empire throughout the Midwest, the industry has been an authority in management, systems development, administration, government, and policy for industry while providing customers with top-quality and safe automobiles that have reshaped modern-day driving capability. With it came people from all over America seeking to take part in the industry's financial gains. It has not been without the hard work of its people who have given, even until death, their lives for the building of cars. Strikes have ranged from sit-ins, sit-downs, walk-outs, slow-downs, sick-outs, work stoppages, and unions have given back to the average blue collar worker what they have given to the automotive industry.

The migration from the southern United States brought many people, including minorities, willing to work for an honest day's pay. Jerry's father was no different. He came to Michigan from Louisiana in the early 1950's and worked for Chevrolet, supporting the family while Jerry's mother stayed home and cared for their five children. Life was better for them in Flint, Michigan, and Jerry grew up determined to get into General Motors. After graduation from high school he did just that. Eventually the future he sought was his. He had the means to get all the material things his heart desired. He worked hard for the money each night in the Buick foundry and overtime was always a given. Third shift was hard. The whole foundry complex was dirty and loud, and there was much lifting of heavy automobile parts but Jerry didn't mind the work. His average paycheck was $975 a week, allowing him to support himself and not be a burden on his family. He could give to his mother who had sacrificed everything for her children over the years. With no wife and children at home he banked the majority of it. He surrounded himself with fine cars, jewelry, clothes, furniture, and several big-screen televisions.

As money rolled in week after week he began to see that there was something missing. The desires of his heart were not met by material wealth and he felt a need for something beyond material furnishings. Restless and unfulfilled, Jerry turned to drugs. Drugs were easy to get as long as money wasn't an obstacle. He became hooked on heroin. Jerry was living large, enjoying the good life. He had it all: women, drugs, cars, money, friends, everything anybody would want. In spite of it all, inside he knew he was headed down a dark road on the fast track to losing it all. His work began to suffer as his supervisor would write him up for late returns to his work station, unexcused absences, missing parts, unsafe work area, and unplanned disappearances during work hours. So on that account he contacted a union representative member who approved treatment in order not to be fired. The union had arranged for treatment of its members who for whatever reason suffered from addictions.

Jerry benefited from the program and committed himself to an after-treatment Narcotics Anonymous meeting each morning after working all night. It was a time to relax and be with like-minded people in similar conditions who had conquered their addition and were prevailing at staying off drugs. He mastered the fear and hollowness he had once felt and began to get past his addiction. It was hard, and he had to stay away from things that would lead him back to heroin addiction.

Then the economy took a downturn and autoworkers were laid off in droves. The local economy in Flint suffered. General Motors' factory workers supported the surrounding economy, and bars, clothing stores, and grocery stores began to lay off personnel. When the offer to transfer to a St. Louis manufacturing plant was extended Jerry jumped on it. He had been laid off for six months and was anxious to get back to work. His move to St. Louis was a chance to change his life, or so he thought. Leaving his family and the support group, Jerry believed he was strong enough to handle his addictive personality and dedicate himself to his work and new life.

St. Louis was a great change for Jerry. He made friends quickly and he had enough seniority to be on first shift. Several months after settling in he met a woman named Sidney at a NA meeting. Sidney was a light-hearted lady who enjoyed life. She was adventurous, intelligent, articulate and encouraging of new ideas. Sidney also worked at the same auto plant but in a different area. Jerry and Sidney began to have lunch together, then they began dating outside the plant. Their relationship grew and over time began to get intensely serious.

On the night they were going to have sex for the first time Sidney told Jerry she had AIDS. He couldn't believe it. He was shocked.

"Why didn't you tell me before now?" Jerry shouted.

She sobbed, "Because I didn't want to lose you, but I couldn't have sex with you without telling you. I didn't want to put you at risk of getting AIDS."

Jerry said nothing, gathered himself, turned, and walked out the door, slamming it shut while she sobbed. Jerry even had brought an engagement ring and planned to ask Sidney to marry him on that night. He felt ready to commit for the first time in his life.

Jerry drove around town thinking about her while looking at the ring he had brought for her. He found himself outside a NA meeting. He parked his car under a tree turned off the motor but couldn't go in. He sat in his car, tears streaming down his cheeks. Music played on the car stereo but Jerry didn't hear it. A friend from the meeting who had come outside to smoke saw him and walked up the car and looked in at him. Jerry was obviously distressed, so his friend got in on the passenger's side and began to talk to him, not realizing what was wrong. He saw the ring in Jerry's hand and asked if she had turned him down.

Jerry shook his head no. "She didn't turn me down. I didn't ask her because she's got AIDS."

"Jerry, I have AIDS too."

Jerry turned and looked at him in shock.

"I got AIDS from my drug-abusing days.

Sharing dirty needles, getting high because that was all that mattered to me. I come here to stay away from that life, those people and the needles. I used heroin like other people drink water. It took over my life. I lost everything: my wife, my children, my home, and my happiness. I couldn't see it, but these meetings made me see. You know the people in there don't play. They tell you about yourself and refuse to let you feel guilty about the wrongs you've done. Instead you take possession, control, and stewardship over past wrongs and move forward, righting your wrongs as best you can. No pity for the pothead here. I have found strength to deal with what I have done to myself. I got AIDS because of what I did not because someone did it to me. It is my fault I have AIDS. I live with that every day of my life."

For the first time Jerry began to see himself. You know I could have AIDS too. I never thought about it. I have never been tested. Maybe I should take a test for AIDS. "Don't judge too quickly Jerry," his NA friend suggested. And with that said the friend got out of the car and went back inside leaving Jerry with much more to think about. Jerry sat for a long time thinking about his life and what he had done. His heroin days rushed back and he thought about getting tested and the possibility of being HIV positive. His head filled with memories of Flint. Before long the meeting let out and people from the meeting began to come out. Jerry looked up and realized he had been sitting under the tree the entire time. He drove home looking at the ring and the circle of happiness he had lost. Jerry was a broken man. Nothing could change the fact that the woman he loved had AIDS.

Unable to sleep he had been awake all night, sitting on his bed and thinking about getting tested, his drug-abusing days, his family, Sidney, and what she must have gone through with her sickness. Guilt overtook him but he couldn't call her.

The next morning at work Jerry was still dazed functioning on autopilot. The morning passed slowly. Before lunch, Sidney walked over to Jerry and put her hand on his shoulder. He turned looked at her and knew he loved her unconditionally. He knew she would remain at the heart of his life. He took her into his arms and apologized for his behavior. Sidney forgave him. Lunch together that day was different. They walked out to the parking lot and sat on a picnic table. Sidney told Jerry that she became infected from using dirty needles and that she had not told anyone, not even discussing it in NA meetings. NA meant so much to both of them, but Sidney could not risk losing the support; besides, she was too scared of rejection by anyone, especially NA, because it had become her saving grace. It had been a heavy burden to carry, not to tell anyone else she had AIDS but she'd carried it. They both knew NA saved lives and had given them a different perspective on themselves and the world.

Her family did not know about her drug abuse. They would not understand and her father would probably disown her. She felt it best never to discuss it with anyone. No one at work knew for fear of retaliation from fellow employees and their employer. She didn't know anyone else at the plant with AIDS. She told Jerry she had gotten a doctor in another town to treat her. She articulated her experience to Jerry with a kind heart, letting him out of the relationship but wanting to remain friends. Sidney's personality shone as bright as the midday sun. Warming his spirit her words comforted him yet horrified him at the same time. Jerry let her talk. She had much to tell him about her life before he walked into it. She was a different person. She had a good job, money, friends, and dope. He smiled inside but kept a straight face, recalling his own past. Jerry sat admiring her strength and courage, understanding her on a different level than before. Sidney didn't know Jerry wanted to marry her.

Lunch soon ended and they returned to their assigned areas, and Sidney smiled to herself that for the first time she told somebody the truth. And the person she told first was the man she loved the most. At the end of his shift Jerry left his area and went to Sidney's area, but she wasn't there. She had left. She went home. Jerry rushed to her house. She answered the door and found him standing with an engagement ring. Sidney began to cry. They flew into each other's arms and he asked her to marry him. "It is right" he said. Sidney couldn't believe he wanted to marry her after what she told him. But Jerry was in love with her and was determined HIV/AIDS could not come between them.

Four years later marriage was agreeing with them. Having a family was planned and discussed with doctors. In agreement, Jerry and Sidney had a beautiful healthy set of triples, two girls and a boy, fifteen months later. Pregnancy was a healthy magical time for her. Their lives were wonderful when Sidney wasn't sick which happened more and more. The babies grew but Sidney grew weaker too. Amy, Annette and Anthony sero-converted to negative and tears of joy overtook Sidney. Jerry grew quiet but his concern showed in his actions and on his face daily. June 15, 36 year old Sidney died of Non-Hodgkin's Lymphoma. Non-Hodgkin's Lymphoma or NHL is a lymphoma made up of B cells and characterized by nodular or diffuse tumors that may appear in the stomach, liver, brain, and bone marrow of persons with HIV. After Kaposi's Sarcoma, NHL is the most common opportunistic cancer in persons with AIDS. Jerry survives with three children.

Mercifully Jerry and Sidney's children could grow up free of the dreaded infection. Not all children of infected parents are so lucky, poor Jimmy was not and he had to suffer ostracism as well as all the trials of his infection. And this was all because of a lack of information that caused Jimmy's friends' parents to tell their children to avoid him. Life can be awfully hard on children with HIV.

I won't play with Jimmy

I won't play with Jimmy
Because Jimmy has got AIDS.

They tried to keep him out of school,
But some judge overturned that rule
Now Jimmy sits behind me, two rows back.
He comes to school like me with books in his back pack.

But Mom said "Don't you play with Jimmy,
Because Jimmy has got AIDS."

The teacher tried to tell us that Jimmy was OK
There really was no reason why he couldn't join our play.
"Just don't get rough," she said
"It could be dangerous if he bled."

But we don't play with Jimmy,
Because Jimmy has got AIDS.

Jimmy used to be my best friend
But Mom said that had to end
Because Jimmy's blood is bad.
"That's so" agreed my Dad.

That's why we don't play with Jimmy,
Because Jimmy has got AIDS.

Sometimes I do feel sad.
It really seems too bad,
That I can't play with Jimmy,
Because Jimmy has got AIDS.

Drinking, Drugs, HIV and My Life
by Aaron Welsh

I was born the middle child and second son to my parents. I had a good childhood and my mom tried to provide all the things I needed. I always felt close to her and she always had a way of making me feel special. My older brother is a year older than I am so we grew up close. My younger sister is a few years younger. We moved to Tennessee when I was about eight. My parents both had jobs at Saturn and my mom was happy. She told us of how our new life was going to be great, so my siblings and I looked forward to the move with expectation. We lived in an apartment for a short while but soon moved to a large white house up on a hill. When I first saw the house I couldn't believe it was ours, but Mom said, "Yes son it's ours." My sister, brother and I were so excited. The house was so big that it had two spare bedrooms and lots of room to play. I loved that house. My parents told me we would never move out of that house and that I would grow up there. I didn't have a problem growing up there because it was a great house. After a few years I finally convinced my parents to let me have my own room. I moved out of the bedroom that I had shared with my brother and into one of the spare rooms. This proved to be a turning point for me. My relationship with my brother began to grow apart as I began to find my independence. Life was good for us in spite of my dad's drinking.

I hated his drinking and could tell my mom's

heart broke each time he said he hadn't been drinking. It was weird that he believed he was getting away with hiding it. My parents separated two or three times, and each time we stayed in the house with mom. The first time they split my dad ended up in a treatment facility and rented a small house out in the country. My mom took us to visit him but I didn't want to go. At some point my dad began cheating on my mom with a woman they worked with at Saturn, and he was drinking a lot. During this time my parents argued all the time. I remember it being a hard time for my Mom. I also remember telling her not to let Dad come back this time. She had already let him come back once by then. She would say, "You all need your dad and I want to do what's best for the family." And then she would take him back. In late 1993 my parents got back together for the third and final time. Things seemed to be going well again and all seemed fine in our house once again.

In 1994 my mom after having surgery, was diagnosed as being HIV positive and so was my father. That completely devastated me and completely changed every aspects of our family. My dad was always an alcoholic. He had been in and out of treatment. Sometimes he'd go to NA meetings. Sometimes he'd take my brother and me with him. I knew about the program from an early age. I didn't know the program but I knew of the program. I started smoking. I didn't smoke a lot just when ever I could steal one from my mom, dad, uncle, or an adult. After a while, around 1996, I was smoking pretty regularly. I kept it from my parents, which wasn't hard to do. Mom seemed sad and us kids tried to cheer her up but she would console us telling us things would get better. They didn't.

My mom told us kids that she was divorcing my dad. My parents got a divorce after my mom put him out for beating her up. Also in '96 my mom lost her job because of HIV. She cried a lot I mean A LOT! I didn't understand what was happening, but stuff wasn't going good in the family and my life seemed to be spinning out of control. My mom stayed sick that year. I was worried a lot. Those were dark times for me, and I push the memories away. Alcohol and AIDS tore our family apart. At the time they told my brother and me about AIDS I knew it kills and believed it was going to kill my mom and dad. I was scared each day I went to school leaving my mom alone. Some days I'd sneak out of class to a phone and call her just to make sure she was still alive. After the divorce I tried weed for the first time. I actually did it to be cool. I was hanging out with a friend at that time, and one of her older guy friends. He was about 20 and I was 13 or 14. He asked me if I ever smoked weed before and I told him yeah because I wanted him to think I had already done that and that I was cool. I got really high, unbelievably high. I ended up getting a little wild. I don't know why but I got in a fight with a big old tree. I loved smoking weed. It was great. It was a release. I didn't care about anything. So I loved it from the very beginning. I actually didn't do it much, maybe once a month or once every two months. Then we ended up moving out of the house where I was growing up. I hated having to move. My mom cried saying "It's happened we've lost the house. I tried to keep it for you kids but I couldn't." We moved to Gatlinburg and I hated it. We moved four miles up in the mountains. It sucked! I started smoking pot in Gatlinburg regularly to numb the growing pain I felt and I got in a lot of trouble at school. I got kicked out of school. That's when I got really into church. The more I used (smoked pot) the more I got into church. Then we moved back to Williamson County and into a house I didn't like. I liked my bedroom but I didn't like the house. I turned sixteen in that house and had my birthday party there. I told my mom I wanted to have a pot party. She absolutely forbade it but I did it anyway. She believed by cutting my guest list she was cutting my exposure to pot. It didn't work. I invited three friends and we got stoned, I mean we got toe up. Soon after that I started using every day: I would use before school, after school at work. I went from job to job to job. No dad in the house, a mom with AIDS, losses, my brother not living with us. All seemed smaller when I used. I wasn't doing well in school. At times I would remember our lives before alcohol and AIDS.

I hated my dad for drinking but one day I decided I was going to get drunk. I went to my mom's room and took a bottle of Bacardi she kept hidden in a closet. I took some and drank it; I felt it and I liked it. I decided I was going to take a little more and ended up getting drunk that night for the first time but I was by myself. I liked getting drunk by myself. I liked getting high by myself. I didn't mind drinking alone, and didn't see anything wrong with drinking hard liquor. That started my drinking spree. I was cool as long as I stayed with the hard stuff. My father was an alcoholic because he drank beer. I was making excuses of reasons why I didn't want to be like him but I was slowly becoming just like him. I ended up drinking hard liquor and then it got to where there wasn't hard liquor around and I wanted to get drunk and there was beer around so I finally ended up drinking beer and I liked it. Beer was so much better than alcohol. Beer became my new thing, my new drug. To drink beer and smoke weed laced with cocaine that was my favorite thing to do. My very, very favorite thing to do, and that's what I would do almost every day. Though mom was in the home, and I knew she cared, spent time with me and all of us kids talking about the ills, drugs, sex, AIDS and everything, she didn't know it was easy for me to get drugs, cause I never had to pay for 'em. The kids were rich and they had money. My friends would buy my drugs for me and I never had a problem with that.

After a while we moved to another house and that's when things got really bad for me. I used pot, pills, alcohol anything I could get my hands on in excess. I'd use every day before school, during school, and after school. I'd use every day before work, during work, and after work. After a while I was working at Backyard Burger, and then my mom told me I could get a job working for her at the agency, WOMEN, she founded in 1996. I thought that was really cool and really wanted to do that, so after a couple months I started working for her. She had no idea. I became a STD HIV/AIDS teen counselor. So I would go to schools and talk to kids and I'd be high, all the while talking to kids about safer sex, drug use, and all this stuff, and I'd be high the whole time. Looking just them I'd tell the high school kids about my using as if it were in the past. I started using heavier and heavier. I stared getting into more pills, acid, mushrooms and things like that. I got into crack cocaine and fell in love with that drug. That was my drug of choice. It started out that I would smoke crack every other Wednesday at school, then it became every Wednesday, and then I started smoking crack a couple times a week. My mom seemed so suspicious of my every move questioning everything. I think she felt something but she had no idea what I was doing. I was a very good actor.

I had my car, money from my job and friends. New Year's Eve 1999 my friend, a guy whom my mother hated, and me went to the train tracks not far from where I lived. We smoked about two or three grams of crack cocaine. After I went back in the house and celebrated the New Year with my family and nobody knew what I had done. Or at least I didn't think they knew about it. I would do sick things like that. I drew away from my family and wanted nothing to do with anyone. Tensions were high with mom. She stayed on my back. I didn't like anybody. I just used people, that's all I ever did, use people for things I wanted. I kept using and using and using. Finally my mother caught me and she told me I had to move out. I was seventeen years old and she told me I had to move out. This was the first time she had ever told me to move. Man, I got scared and began talking my way out of having to move out. No way was I movin'. She changed her mind and I didn't have to move out so from then on her threats of forcing me out were just weak talk that didn't really mean anything. I just thought she was trying to exercise some power trip over me, or something like that. I kept using and using and things got much worse. She ended up kicking me out for a second time. This time I had to go. Moving from friend to friend until their parents caught on made eating, showering and even having clean clothes hard to come by. I had been in and out of juvenile court and on probation since I was about thirteen years old. I got arrested again for violating curfew. My mom had a house curfew but that didn't mean much. I had been arrested for the same thing four or five times, and she was sick of it. She was sick of me getting arrested, sick of having to deal with going to court and sick of picking me up from jail after another weekend stay. She was completely fed up.

Turning seventeen I was still using hard and heavy, still hanging out with my drug-using buddies, and one thing led to another and I was arrested again. I got put on probation again. I was going to have to be on probation for two years but then I turned eighteen and the judge told me I was too old for his court and gave me a stern lecture. The judge dismissed all charges and let me off. I didn't have a problem with that but told myself I was going to be good from then on, and for a while I tried to be good. I kept using but tried to be good. Me and using: I can never be good when I'm using no matter how hard I try. So I turned eighteen and two weeks after they let me off juvenile probation I got arrested again but this time I was arrested as an adult. I got arrested with the same guy with whom I smoked crack. We got pulled over for window tint and not wearing our seat belts. They searched the car, searched me, and searched him. They found a quarter pound of weed on me, an ounce of cocaine on him as well as an opened bottle of alcohol in the car so we went to jail. I went to court for that and got put on probation with a sentence of 11 months 29 days. With that sentence hanging over my head I did two weekends in jail. After that I was never going to get in trouble again. Hey, the judge said next time I was in jail 11 months and 29 days. I had been to jail and didn't like it. I had had it. I was on probation, I didn't want to go to jail, and I was fed up with it. About three weeks later my mom went out of town.

I decided I was going to have a little party. My brother had come back to stay with us. Feeling responsible, I guess, he didn't like the fact that we were drinking and doing drugs in the house so he called the cops. Just before the cops came I found out what he had done and I ran out of the house and hid and the other people partying with me ran out of the house. The cops didn't find us so we got away. In my mind I thought everything was all right so the next night, with my mother still gone, I decided to have another party with the same group of friends. But this time I unplugged the phone so my brother couldn't call the cops. My brother went to the nearby gas station and called the cops again. He also called my mother on her cell phone in her hotel room and told her what I was doing in her house but at the time I didn't know he had told her. My brother's call to the cops brought them again but I had decided I was going to run again. This time I didn't get away. I was so high and drunk I stumbled over myself, unable to stand up. I ran to the gas station to get cigarettes and they popped me at the gas station. It really sucked. I didn't know what to do.

The cops took me back to my house and they called my mom's cell phone. They asked her if she wanted me to go to jail or just leave me at the house. Mom said, "Take him to jail." That kicked me. I had this huge resentment toward my mom for doing that to me. So I went to jail. We had all kinds of drugs in the house that they didn't find. I called my brother from jail and he told me the cops found the drugs with the assistance of drug-sniffing dogs. I couldn't believe the cops brought dogs in my house. While in jail I kept thinking I was screwed so I devised a plan to run away. My brother hocked his TV to post my bail, but I was so mad at him I didn't care about him or his TV. After getting out of jail my buddy and I decided to run away. His parents were rich and said that they were going to buy us a houseboat and we were going to live on the houseboat. His parents were cool like that and it sounded like a plan to me. I just wanted to run from all the charges because I knew I was going to be doing some time. At the last minute my buddy backed out and my mom wouldn't let me come back home, so I had nowhere to live. I was staying a few nights at one friend's house then a few nights at another's. Then I went to stay with a friend who had the party house. This was the house where everyone would get high, drunk, and get laid. There you could do whatever you wanted to. This kid's mother lived there but she didn't care. She would buy the alcohol. I lived there with him for about a week or two. At that time I didn't see a reason to live. I didn't see a reason to keep going. I felt alone and unloved, so I ended up doing a lot of drugs. The move had been really hard on both of us. I seemed to have a don't care attitude because everything I loved or wanted was taken away and in my heart I knew my mom would die soon of AIDS so why care about anything, so I decided then and there that I was going to kill myself. I went back to get high at the house where I was staying and did a whole bunch of drugs, got really drunk, I mean super high and then I took 240 aspirins. I had seen in a movie that if you take over 30 aspirin your heart can't handle it so that's what I did. I took it all and fell asleep. It was the weirdest thing when I woke up: I thought I was dead but I wasn't. When I woke it felt like I had never breathed before. I took that first breath and it was like I was breathing life back into my body. It was amazing. After that I threw up everywhere and got really sick. Everybody was asking what was wrong, but I didn't tell them because I knew they would make me go to the hospital and I didn't want to go the hospital. They found the empty aspirin bottle. The kid's mother called my mom and told her that I had taken a large amount of aspirin. The kid's mother didn't know exactly how many I had taken but remembered the bottle having being full. My mother must have told her to call the ambulance, 'cause before I knew it three men were putting me on a bed and taking my limp body out the door into the night air. I felt as if I were floating. It all seems so hazy. I just wanted to die.

I spent four days in the hospital. My heart stopped while I was in the emergency room. My mom, brother, and sister came to see me the next day. I could see the worry on my mom's face. Pale and drawn, she cried when she first saw me. I was angry with my brother for calling the cops and wanted nothing to do with him, but my mom scolded me so I never said anything mean to him. My sister made jokes and nervously explored the hospital room. While I was in the hospital I decided I didn't want to live the way I was. My life had no meaning, no purpose, and no source. My whole life was built around drugs. Everything I did was centered on drugs; either using drugs, getting drugs, or using people to get drugs. Everything I did was to get drugs, everything. I truly did not want to live that way any more but it was hard. My parent's HIV status and divorce had taken away my will to live, and, now, finally, it was back. On my fourth day at the hospital I underwent an assessment and was discharged to the Cumberland Heights Youth In-patient Treatment Program. I agreed to the in treatment thirty-day youth program because I needed something. Shortly after arriving at Cumberland Heights we were told that not even 10 percent of us would make it. There were less than ten new kids entering into the program with me. So less than ten percent was pretty much nobody. To this day I am the only one out of the group who has not relapsed, gone back out, or stayed out. I've been close so many times. To live like this is hard. To not do something I can do so well. I was always so much better than everybody else at using drugs. I could do so much more than everyone and everybody thought that was cool. I began using drugs at age thirteen because it was something to do.

Meetings have become a part of my life and are my daily reprieve refuge and relief. I prefer AA meetings to all other meetings. My Cumberland Heights experience gave me the base in sobriety. I am about a year clean rooted in the 12-step program, completed one year of probation without getting in trouble and am still working for my mom at Women On Maintaining Education and Nutrition, doing the same job but now with my heart, soul and experience. I set up youth meetings for teen addicts to come to. I still do school outreach, but now I can do it with a clear head. It's a completely different feeling. My mom is still around and I've come to understand that she is living with AIDS and time with her is more precious than anything.

Aaron Welsh, who wrote this painfully honest account of the devastating effects of HIV on himself and his family, is now 23. He continues to work as a youth peer counsellor and educator at WOMEN, the community organization founded by his mother. He has now been clean for several years and is the proud father of a baby daughter, Cayla Faith.

This story was first published in "The Lilypad," Fall issue, 2005.

Aaron - Back from the Abyss

Despair combined with drugs - a recipe for disaster,
A combination well night impossible to master.
He tried to kill himself, but, thank God, failed,
But he could not escape from being jailed.

He got a wake-up call that shook him to the core.
The drugs, the booze, the sex just could not help him any more
But in spite of all the things to which his body he subjected
His good luck held and he was not infected.

Now his karma he's redeeming,
Acting honestly, no longer scheming,
But speaking truth to people just like him,
Young people on society's outer rim.

How great a turnaround was this;
He pulled back up from the edge of the abyss.

Tommy Morris - A Balanced Life

If you met Tommy, I am sure you would like him. He's good looking, talented and friendly. You would probably assume that he was Chinese from his appearance but ethnically, as his name might suggest, he is really a bit of a mix. Tommy is gay and comes from Los Angeles. I have known him for fifteen years or more and I have seen no changes or deterioration in his health, not that I know anything about his T cell count or other important factors. I think he has kept well for several reasons. He lives a disciplined life. He has had the same partner ever since I met him. I believe he is disciplined over eating, drinking, exercise, and all the other things that any other health conscious male would be. Tommy has a great spirit and this no doubt is a major factor.

I mentioned that he was talented. He plays the piano and sings well and he has been a successful actor, though he complains that it is difficult for him as a man who looks like an oriental Asian to get parts that do not demand skills in the martial arts or that cast him in anything other than some minor role such as a waiter in a Chinese or Thai restaurant. His abilities deserve more than this.

I know that when Tommy was offered a managerial position in a small company in in New England he let the president of the company know that he was HIV positive. The president appreciated Tommy's honesty but never divulged the information to any of Tommy's coworkers. Whether any of them knew of his health status I cannot say, but if they did it could only be because Tommy had told them himself. Presumably they did know that he was gay. Tommy was a popular member of staff and some of his coworkers have kept in touch with him, long after he and his partner moved away from New England.

In one respect Tommy was very lucky, he has always had insurance coverage that paid for his anti-retroviral drugs. This has no doubt been one of the contributory reasons why Tommy has been able to continue his life as a productive member of society despite his infection. In fact Tommy is the living proof that given the necessary support and understanding there is no reason why a person infected with the HIV virus cannot live a useful and satisfying life for many years. They just need to be given the chance.

Don't think that I am saying that HIV can be taken lightly. Although Tommy has dealt so well with his life as an HIV positive person, the fact is that it is a terrible and incurable infection that can lead to cancers and other major medical problems even for those who do have the support, medication and understanding they need. What I am saying is that if everyone infected could be given the support, the medicines, and the understanding, many more than at present could go on for years living useful and reasonably satisfying lives, contributing to society rather than becoming burdens to themselves, their families and to society. It is really up to the rest of us to see that this can happen.

(Some names in this piece have been changed.)

Positive man, lucky man

Although I have this virus,
We should never let it mire us
In a desperate swamp of worry.
Relax, live every minute, what's the hurry?

I keep my body fit and mind alert
Even when it does begin to hurt.
I enjoy the music and the song.
That always helps me get along.

I take exercise but do not strain.
It helps me to forget the pain.
I've so much to be thankful for
And every day I find there's more.

I've a faithful partner who really cares.
I've loyal friends who give themselves no airs.
In spite of my infection I have a life that's good
And I dearly wish that all the others could.

I've got good health insurance and I'm very grateful.
It's so wrong that other are deprived. It's hateful.
I can go on living in a happy, productive way,
While others are just left to rot their lives away.

I know that I am lucky and can live a life that's good.
Even with HIV, it's possible. Understood?
But for people that's poor and black, it's not the same.
And this discrimination is humanity's greatest shame.

Ashley Maria - Angel waiting for the Light

I will tell you so you will never forget when you next see one of the ambassadors of the next generation. Ashley Maria is our next generation and her time along with those to come has indeed inherited AIDS from our generation. Ashley is eight years old and likes to tell people that her birthday is November 23. She has lived well below the poverty level her entire eight years. Ashley was born with AIDS.

Most people have no idea what life has been like for this beautiful child. Ashley is a child whose heart is filled with love, and her arms surround others with hope. With upturned face her eyes sparkle like big brown saucers. This baby (for she is a baby) has compassion for everyone she knows.

At eight years old Ashley remains in the third grade, and is unable to attend school regularly due to reccurring illness. Though she communicates very well, her educational level and developmental and social skills are limited. She hurts in one way or the other constantly. She knows little about a normal nuclear family but longs for the family life she sees on television. Her entire life has been spent living with her grandmother, who is very old and has her own health problems, and her mother, who is ill with full-blown AIDS. Ashley's mother became infected after receiving a blood transfusion in her sixth month of pregnancy. Her mother sits helplessly at her bedside looking at the beautiful angel that is Ashley. Ashley has seen her mother's tears. Ashley knows not a day without AIDS, this baby has been poked, prodded, injected, infected, hospitalized for months at a time, and has a medical history longer than she is tall. She has been near death twice since I have known her. This is a child with AIDS. She has seen and spoken to God. Her description of God took my breath away. Imagine seeing God through a child's eyes.

Your busy life is much different than hers. Her life has more to do with survival and getting through the next series of always-scheduled tests. While you are busy with work and getting your healthy children tucked safely away at school, Ashley might be sitting in a waiting room, throwing up last night's meal, which had to be forced down her, or she's so tired she can't get out of bed period. Years of waiting rooms, hospital emergency rooms, infectious disease specialists, and nurses have educated her about the future she now struggles with. These things are hard for her to comprehend; she's heard the adults talking about patients and family members whom they've buried and loved ones who are in severely advanced stages of the same disease that brings her to this place.

Later while we are getting off work and retrieving healthy children from a day of learning, socializing and interacting with others their age, Ashley lies still because movement brings more pain. She hurts most days for one reason or another. Her arm gets infected from the needles and several times a month her pick line must be replaced. The port she had in her chest February 3 was surgically removed November 1. She is taking so many medications that a shunt had to be placed in her chest because some of the drugs helping her stay alive taste awful. Forcing Ashley to take them is more than her sick mother can do. An extensive blood test revealed a bacterial infection had surrounded the area above her left breast. At times it becomes difficult for Ashley to speak because her lungs often restrict her inhalations. Her legs are like toothpicks and give way, causing her more pain. She's been confined to a wheelchair, to bed, and she's been confined to her family's two bedroom apartment. She has to stay away from others during cold and flu season, because she is more concerned about getting your germs than you are about getting hers. She is confined by AIDS.

To be a child one must be able to talk on the phone, hang out at the mall, and trash parental attempts to control a young life. Young Ashley has not been able to do those simple things. Instead her friends are adults who always tell her to be sure and take her medicine. Several of them have made empty promises about future events that come to pass. In spite of her disease she longs for the day when she's free of the chains of AIDS. Ashley no longer shows interest in sustaining her earthly life with medication. Instead she looks for the light, the embracing light she has seen and now wishes to become a part of.

Children are living epistles that stand as evidence to the future that the past has made some level of contribution. Your children, my children, everyone's children are the literary work of hope yet to come. Ashley will not test the limits of her destiny; instead her destiny is locked in AIDS.

Ashley Maria succumbed to an AIDS related illness January 28th. Her grandmother died a month prior. Ashley's mother is frail having lost well over half her body weight. She lives in shelters, on the streets doing drugs, trading sex for drugs to support her addiction. Do you suppose she tells her sex partner she's infected and has full blown AIDS?

Poor Kids - But it's not my fault!

I know what happens to these kids. It's such a shame.
But don't look at me so pointedly, I'm not to blame.
Their mothers were all HIV infected
And now these poor infected children are neglected.

But, thank God, that's not my problem, although I sympathize.
Something should be done, no one denies.
Places like India and Africa are far away.
Their governments should do more, I would say.

And as for those kids in the ghettoes of our city,
I don't see how I could help them, more's the pity.
You say they're my little sisters, little brothers
And I should care about them and their mothers.

What do you mean?
I act responsibly and I've stayed clean.
It's up to those responsible to sort these problems out.
Don't look at me. I have no position and no clout.

Such arguments and attitudes won't get us anywhere.
Things only can get better when by actions we show we really care.

Sonny - Orphaned by AIDS

Women have historically been considered the primary caregivers of children. In the past women stayed home while men financially supported the family. More recently single parenting has become a societal norm, and additionally many women have elected to raise children alone, even eliminating the man entirely with artificial insemination or other methods. Divorce rates have increased and the numbers of homes that are fatherless have skyrocketed.

Social service and state organizations have recognized nonpayment of child support as a social injustice and have begun to enforce deadbeat father's responsibilities. Men have also been ostracized from homes and forced into positions that do not allow them to see their children. There are men who do care about their children and want to be a part of their lives even if the marriage doesn't work. But what does this mean for the children? Broken homes and shattered memories of what family once meant to a child, have often been replaced by mothers who try to be moms/workers/housekeepers/pillars of society while accomplishing little for themselves. What does this mean for the children?

Sonny, an only child, is a very confused ten-year-old. His dad had left home in an ambulance with big flashing lights last year. Nancy, his mother, told Sonny that Daddy was sick and that the nice people were going to take good care of him and that he should be home soon. But Daddy never came back, and

Sonny couldn't figure out why. During the week of the funeral neighbors and family members began to talk, whispering, "He died of AIDS. I wonder if she's infected. I wonder if the boy has it." Nancy and her HIV negative son were left to deal with the shame of disease. Sonny only wanted his family back. He wanted things to be the way they used to be when the family ate dinner together and when Daddy and Mommy tucked him in bed at night.

Sonny's mother died of an AIDS-related infection six months later, but Sonny still asks where she is and when she will come to take him home? Too young to understand, Sonny was not allowed to see her while she lay dying in the hospital. His rage, frustration, and emotional outbursts have become common. The child has not only lost his father and mother, but people have begun telling him his mother died of AIDS. AIDS stole Sonny's parents and left him orphaned, discriminated against, and frightened.

As the numbers of orphaned children continues to escalate in this country, the children who are left behind are in desperate need of new homes and extensive support. Without legal protection an orphan's situation becomes even more precarious. New guardians often cannot obtain immediate financial and medical benefits for the child or even enroll the child in school.

Without proper support, fear, secrecy, and embarrassment can affect a child's mind. Children orphaned by AIDS are forced to deal with things they are often unable to process, let alone understand. Inattentiveness, disruptive behavior, and poor academic skills follow children orphaned by AIDS. All things associated with school - relationships with other children, teachers and class work - suffer. Good intentions can backfire as children withdraw and retreat inward. Children orphaned by AIDS blame themselves and harbor deep anger toward others and themselves. With love, children orphaned by AIDS can be encouraged to live again. This is a national mental health crisis and no one is paying attention!

Sonny lives in a well-kept orphanage while waiting to be adopted. He continues to receive intensive mental support but concerns for how long managed care will bless his treatment remains utmost in the minds of the already drained health care specialists working at the orphanage. Managed care and mental health services are currently at odds. While managed care determines the length of services, children in need of mental health services are left to figure out how they must deal with the multiple issues surrounding death. Along with all the changes Sonny and other children face, there is the issue of adoption. Adoption and AIDS are two words that are hard for any ten-year-old to grasp. Placement of children whose parents die of AIDS is a difficult placement, but that is changing.

Much that cries out in me cries for the children. Infected or affected, with parents or without parents children are certainly in need of maintenance, love, education and security. Our country is in a delayed state of evolution with regards to HIV education. We need to focus on prevention education, through the many AIDS organizations and support groups. There is a great deal of money given to charitable AIDS organizations, and we all know about the famous "red ribbon." Even with all this AIDS continues to spread. AIDS continues to destroy families. AIDS continues to kill.

It is clear from some of the stories in this book (for example, Cheryl's story), that because of the way HIV is normally spread, (i.e. through sexual contact, particularly unprotected sex, or by using unsterilized hypodermic needles) there is very often a sense of shame attached to becoming infected. The infected person is suspected of promiscuity, infidelity or drug addiction. In addition, owing to the fear of, and lack of understanding about, the disease, the infected person is shunned. So they keep quiet and try to hide their health status. This in turn often means that they do not seek the treatment and support that is available. So their condition deteriorates rapidly. In some cases they may unintentionally or negligently infect others.

A Last Piece of Advice

If you find you've been infected
Or have some problem you've suspected
Might be HIV,
Can't you see
You simply must
Confide in someone you can trust.
Your doctor is the obvious choice
And if the doc is sympathetic, not judgmental, then rejoice,
For now you can begin to get
The treatment and supporting net,
Which you will surely need.
Part of your burden will be lifted off your back
For now, although infected, you are on the track
That leads to survival and a worthwhile existence.

You can go on living with persistence
Even enjoying life and all it brings
Upon its wings
Until the time comes that must befall
That life will end, as it does for all.
So I beg you please, heed this advice
And don't go lonely, turned to ice.

What Now?

Well, what now? We've said what we have had to say.
I guess it's your turn now, O.K.?
If we have made you think a little more
And made you want to take a stand in this global war
Against this scourge, our aim will be fulfilled.
If we've called you to action, we'll be thrilled.
You can contribute in so many ways.
This work will go on till we end our days.
Funds are needed as one form of support
But with money alone this war cannot be fought.
We need to educate our neighbors, help them understand
How deeply HIV and AIDS affect our land.
AIDS is not a punishment from God.
(If he would vent his punishment on kids, he must be very odd!)
In this world there's just one family, the human one.
Lets help each other till the work is done.

Catherine *Ian*

Appendix

Adolescents, AIDS and Rural America

HIV infection and AIDS is an increasingly serious health threat for adolescents in the United States. The epidemic is shifting to young people, with one quarter of all new infections estimated to occur in persons between the age thirteen and twenty. Two Americans under the age of twenty become infected with HIV every hour of each day. The impact of AIDS in our country is increasing in small communities. Rural AIDS cases rose from five percent of the total AIDS cases in 1990 to more than seven percent in 1997.

Rural America is not immune to HIV infection no matter how much it is denied. Denial can be fatal. Numbers of new infections are multiplying at a rapid rate and the AIDS epidemic has become increasingly dangerous as it spreads through rustic America. The CDC reported a 5.3 percent increase in AIDS where residency is less than 500,000. A need for epidemiological research and public health intervention to determine why HIV infection continues to be increasing in small cities and rural areas is crucial. Educational programs must be developed based upon the unique characteristics of rural communities, where, generally, everyone knows everyone else. These programs must protect the privacy of its participants. The programs must be realistic, and up-to-date and directly impact adolescents. In addition programs must address all the issues neighboring HIV infection, including STD education, sex education, and abstinence education.

Abstinence is possible.

Peer pressure, immaturity, drugs, and alcohol play a role in increased rates of HIV infection among high school and college students in rural and urban areas. Students in rural areas are less likely to take precautions against acquiring HIV when under the influence of mind-altering substances and more likely to give in to peer pressure to do things they might not otherwise do if not under the influence of drugs. Date rape occurs in rural America at unmarked rates because females do not report rape in many cases. Small-town lifestyles where most everyone knows their neighbor is also a contributing factor.

Nowadays there is much more than unwanted pregnancies to be concerned about when having welcomed or unwelcomed sex. Rural America has a phenomenon called the illusion of unique vulnerability according to a study done in 1988. This phenomenon is affecting the judgment of negative incidences. HIV/AIDS will have a great impact on the next generation of adults in rural cities and town.

Since this disease generally does not show its ill effects until years after the antibodies are detected, many adolescents and young adults will not become ill from HIV until later in life. Therefore it is imperative that adolescents and young adults in rural America learn more than just the facts about HIV/AIDS. Prevention skills based on behavior and an understanding of why they chose to put themselves at risk must be included in education.

In 1997 African-Americans accounted for close to

58 percent of the pediatric AIDS cases in the United States. Despite the declines in mother-to-baby transmission from using AZT during pregnancy, labor, delivery, and for the first six months after birth, the majority of babies born with AIDS continued to occur among African-Americans. In addition, in 1997 African-American children accounted for 60 percent of the total number of children with parents with AIDS. The severe impact among African-American children indicates the need for enormous efforts to prevent infection among African-American women and to reach larger numbers of HIV positive pregnant women with early prenatal care and preventive treatment.

Are you HIV+?

* Get tested; use anonymous testing if you feel it necessary but get tested.

* Learn your options and line up your support. Support systems are extremely important.

* Get a mental health professional you trust involved.

* If you are HIV positive or have AIDS maximize your health.

* Get a full immune health workup and a complete physical, and become informed.

* Get and ask to see your baseline CD4 (T cell) and viral load test, repeat quarterly.

* Keep careful records.

* Get active in your health care and take control.

* Understand the numbers, trends, medications and medical system.

* When choosing medications know all you can about reactions to other medications including over-the-counter products (drug interactions).

* Lean about preventive treatment against PCP

(Pneumocystis carinii pneumonia) and other OIs.

* Learn about nutrition and what works for you through a nutrition specialist and/or your doctor.

* Consider more or less aggressive antiviral regimen if necessary.

* Remain on any preventative treatments you have started for at least six months.

* If on HIV/AIDS medications take them as prescribed.

* Learn about holistic approaches to health care (massage therapy, meditation, herbs, inner peace, mind/body connection).

AIDS Defining Conditions

The Centers for Disease Control and Prevention (CDC) defines an HIV+ person with a CD4 cell count of 200 or less as having AIDS. The CDC has also developed a list of more than 20 opportunistic infections (OIs) that are considered AIDS-defining conditions (see below). If you have HIV and one or more of these OIs, you have a diagnosis of AIDS.

This list comes from a government report and contains medical terms. If you have any questions, contact a treatment educator at a local AIDS service organization or call an AIDS information line such as the Project Inform National HIV/AIDS Treatment Hotline at 800-822-7422.

Candidiasis of bronchi, trachea, or lungs
Candidiasis, esophageal
Cervical cancer, invasive
Coccidioidomycosis, disseminated or extrapulmonary
Cryptococcosis, extrapulmonary
Cryptosporidiosis, chronic intestinal (greater than 1 month's duration)
Cytomegalovirus disease (other than liver, spleen, or nodes)
Cytomegalovirus retinitis (with loss of vision
Encephalopathy, HIV-related
Herpes simplex: chronic ulcer(s) (greater than 1 month's duration); or bronchitis, pneumonitis, or esophagitis

Histoplasmosis, disseminated or extrapulmonary
Isosporiasis, chronic intestinal (greater than 1 month's duration)
Kaposi's sarcoma
Lymphoma, Burkitt's (or equivalent term)
Lymphoma, immunoblastic (or equivalent term)
Lymphoma, primary, of brain
Mycobacterium avium complex or M. kansasii, disseminated or extrapulmonary
Mycobacterium tuberculosis, any site (pulmonary or extrapulmonary) Mycobacterium, other species or unidentified species, disseminated or extrapulmonary
Pneumocystis carinii pneumonia
Pneumonia, recurrent
Progressive multifocal leukoencephalopathy
Salmonella septicemia, recurrent
Toxoplasmosis of brain
Wasting syndrome due to HIV

ISBN 141207662-5

9 781412 076623

Made in United States
Troutdale, OR
11/03/2026

56847414R00066